I0500521

THE ULTIMATE
KIDNEY TRANSPLANT
SMOOTHIE RECIPES
COOKBOOK

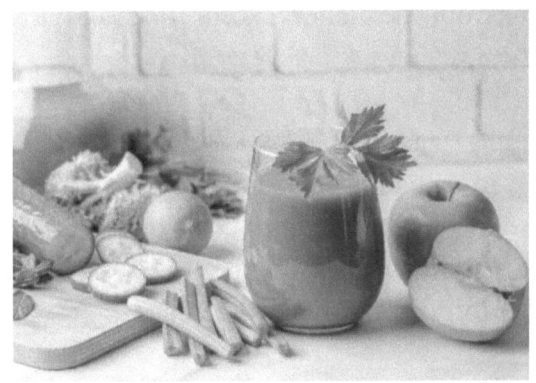

Discover Quick And Tasty Kidney-Friendly
Smoothie Recipes For Kidney Transplant
Patient And Manage Renal Health Effectively

Kathleen Scribner

Copyright © [Kathleen Scribner], [2023]

Read more books by Kathleen Scribner by visiting:
https://www.amazon.com/author/skathleen234

All rights reserved. No part of this book may be reproduced or transmitted in any form or by any means, electronic or mechanical, including photocopying, recording, or by any information storage and retrieval system, without permission in writing from the author, except for brief quotations in critical reviews or articles.

The author has taken great care to present accurate and up-to-date information; however, the author and publisher do not assume any responsibility for errors or omissions or for the use or interpretation of the information contained herein.

TABLE OF CONTENTS

INTRODUCTION

CHAPTER ONE: KIDNEY TRANSPLANT SMOOTHIE

The Benefits of Kidney Transplant Smoothie

Tips to Kidney Transplant Smoothie

40 Tasty And Easy Nutritious Smoothie Recipes For Kidney Transplant Patient

1. Berry Blast Smoothie

2. Cucumber Mint Cooler

3. Spinach and Banana Delight

4. Apple Pie Smoothie

5. Tropical Twist

6. Avocado Banana Smoothie

7. Carrot Cake Smoothie

8. Peachy Green Smoothie

9. Cherry Almond Delight

10. Pomegranate Berry Smoothie

11. Almond Butter Banana Smoothie

12. Spinach and Pineapple Green Smoothie

13. Oatmeal Cookie Smoothie

14. Watermelon Mint Cooler

15. Raspberry Almond Protein Smoothie

16. Blueberry Spinach Smoothie

17. Carrot Ginger Delight

18. Mango Banana Coconut Smoothie

19. Blackberry Walnut Bliss

20. Strawberry Cucumber Refresher

21. Papaya Passion Smoothie
22. Banana Walnut Breakfast Smoothie
23. Kiwi Lime Cooler
24. High-Protein Smoothie with Peaches
25. Vanilla Almond Smoothie
26. Blueberry Oatmeal Smoothie
27. Cherry Coconut Dream
28. Mango Spinach Green Smoothie
29. Raspberry Peach Bliss
30. Lemon Berry Zest
31. Green Apple Cinnamon Smoothie
32. Banana Blueberry Chia Smoothie
33. Spinach and Pineapple Protein Boost
34. Carrot-Orange Sunshine Smoothie
35. Simple Protein Smoothie with Pineapple
36. Smoothie with Fruit
37. Protein Shake with Mixed Berries
38. Pineapple Mint Refresher
39. High-Protein Strawberry Smoothie
40. Mixed Berry Spinach Delight
CONCLUSION

INTRODUCTION

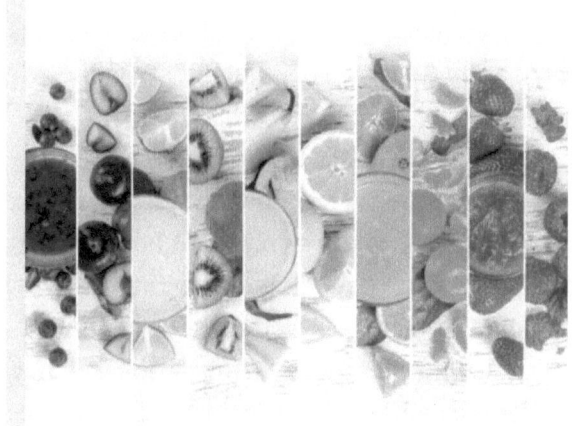

Say you could imagine the sensation of being born again. A second shot at life, a renewed sense of optimism coursing through your body. This is the tale of Joe, a kidney transplant recipient who dealt with the difficulties of long-term renal failure, much as a lot of other patients do. Joe's journey started with something as basic as a smoothie, and it ended with a miraculous turnaround in his life.

Kidney illness has been Joe's reality for many years. It was an unending struggle, an ongoing tug-of-war for his survival. He could no longer remember how many times he had seen doctors, how many times he had to follow rigorous diet plans, and how much exhaustion seemed to follow him everywhere. He felt as if time was passing quickly and that he was getting closer to the edge of hopelessness every day.

Then Joe had a kidney transplant, which turned his life around and provided the much-needed lifeblood. It was as if a glimmer of hope had broken through the ominous clouds hanging above him. Although the transplant procedure went well, Joe knew that his ordeal was far from done. A new set of difficulties surfaced in the post-transplant period, such as eating limitations to protect his just donated kidney.

Joe's diet needed to be adjusted to preserve renal function at its best, which entailed limiting his consumption of phosphorus and potassium. Smoothies were a key component of the notion of kidney-friendly diets and drinks that his healthcare staff presented to him.

Smoothies have become more than simply a delicious treat for Joe and many other kidney transplant patients. They developed it as an essential instrument for taking back control of their health. Smoothies that are suitable for kidneys are made to be tasty, nourishing, and easy on the kidneys. They don't overwork the important organ since they are poor in potassium and phosphorus.

These smoothies combine ingredients like yogurt, almonds, leafy greens, and fresh fruits to create a symphony of tastes. They provide people like Joe with sustenance and support while they rebuild their lives, serving as more than simply a means to an end. They are a celebration of life, wellness, and the pleasure of indulging in a delightful and revitalizing beverage.

We want to provide you with a range of tastes and alternatives in this selection of kidney transplant smoothie recipes that you may enjoy and customize to fit your own dietary requirements. We are excited about serving as a resource for those who have started their own post-transplant journey and are looking for ways to feed themselves that are fulfilling and healthy.

The amazing journey that Joe and many others like him have taken is now available to you, one drink at a time, via these recipes, whether you're a kidney transplant patient, caregiver, or just interested in preserving kidney health.

CHAPTER ONE: KIDNEY TRANSPLANT SMOOTHIE

The Benefits of Kidney Transplant Smoothie

Smoothies for kidney transplantation may seem sophisticated, but they are really super beverages that are very beneficial to your health, particularly if you have had a kidney transplant. Let's examine the many advantages of these delicious and nourishing drinks.

1. Kidney-Friendly Goodness: Your newly transplanted kidney needs a little more attention after surgery. Smoothies that are suitable for kidneys are made with your kidneys in mind. They don't overdo it on elements like potassium and phosphorus, which your kidneys can have trouble with.

2. Easy to Digest: Smoothies like this are gentle on the stomach. They act as a soft embrace for your inside organs, facilitating your body's absorption of healthy nutrients including minerals and vitamins.

3. Tasty and Enjoyable: Smoothies with kidney transplants are not just health benefits—they taste great! They are available in a variety of tastes, ranging from nutty to creamy to fruity, so you can enjoy the flavor and look after your kidneys at the same time.

4. Nutrient Boost: They're packed with nutrients that your body needs. Ingredients like fresh fruits, leafy greens, yogurt, and nuts provide your body with vitamins and energy.

5. Keeps You Hydrated: It's critical to stay hydrated, particularly after a kidney transplant. Smoothies with kidney transplants often include a high water content, which might help you reach your daily hydration targets.

6. Convenient and Quick: Hectic schedules? Not an issue. These smoothies are quick and simple to prepare, making them a great option for those who are often on the move.

7. Supports Your Recovery: Kidney transplant smoothies can be a part of your recovery plan. They give you a tasty way to nourish your body, which will make you feel stronger and more energized as you heal.

8. Versatile and Customizable: Smoothies may be customized to your preferences and dietary requirements. To customize them to your specifications, swap out or add ingredients.

9. A Source of Joy: Smoothies with kidney transplants might add a little joy to your day. It resembles a modest celebration of wellness.

Smoothies are a great complement to your post-transplant journey, to put it briefly. They are a delightful, nourishing, and kidney-friendly method of caring for your health. These smoothies provide a quick and pleasurable route to wellbeing, regardless of whether you've had a kidney transplant or just want to promote kidney health.

Tips to Kidney Transplant Smoothie

Smoothies made with kidney transplant ingredients may be a delightful and healthful method to promote kidney function. Consult your healthcare provider and choose ingredients with reduced potassium and phosphorus content to get the most out of these smoothies. To get more nutrients without taxing the kidneys, use leafy greens like spinach and kale and fruits like apples, berries, and peaches. Eat in moderation and stay away from foods rich in potassium, such as oranges and bananas.

Take into account non dairy milk substitutes such as coconut or almond milk, which are often reduced in phosphorus. Supplemental nutrition should be used with caution as it may contain excessive concentrations of certain minerals. Make sure the protein powder you add to your smoothies is kidney-friendly. Try different combinations of fruits, veggies, and liquids to make your meals unique and in line with your nutritional requirements.

Smoothies might help you achieve a balance in your regular fluid consumption. Enjoy in moderation since general health depends on a balanced diet that includes a range of foods. Keep a regular eye on your blood levels of phosphorus and potassium so you may modify your diet as necessary. To monitor your eating patterns and how they impact your health, keep a food journal. Check nutritional labels and internet resources to stay up to date on the nutritional makeup of various components.

To make sure your kidney transplant smoothies continue to support your health and well-being, keep in regular contact with your healthcare physician or nutritionist. Keep in mind that your dietary demands may alter over time.

40 Tasty And Easy Nutritious Smoothie Recipes For Kidney Transplant Patient

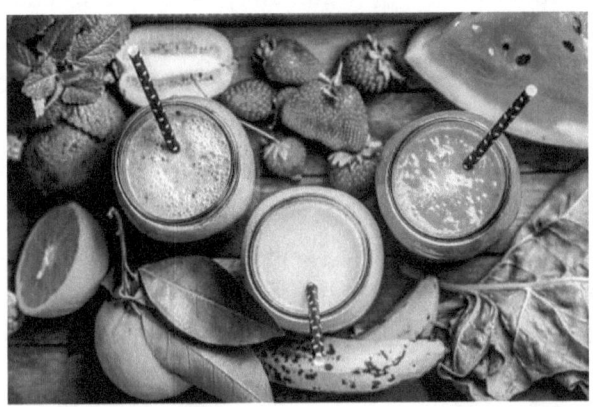

1. Berry Blast Smoothie

Ingredients:

- 1/2 cup of blueberries
- 1/2 cup of strawberries
- 1/2 cup of unsweetened yogurt
- 1/2 cup of water
- 1 tablespoon of honey (optional)

Instructions:

Strawberries and blueberries must be well cleaned for these recipes. After that, the ingredients are blended together with the addition of one tablespoon of honey for sweetness. The berries are then thoroughly mixed into the smoothie and churned until smooth. Depending on taste, additional honey or water may be added to change the sweetness or thickness. You may enjoy the Berry Blast Smoothie as a cool, kidney-friendly treat by serving it in a glass with fresh berries on top. Berries may be used fresh or frozen in this recipe, and water can be added or subtracted to change the thickness. A spoonful of flaxseed meal may be added for extra fiber and good fats. The recipe may be modified to fit personal tastes and requirements.

2. Cucumber Mint Cooler

Ingredients:

- 1/2 cucumber, peeled and sliced
- A handful of fresh mint leaves
- 1/2 cup of plain yogurt
- 1/2 cup of water
- 1 teaspoon of honey (optional)

Instructions:

This recipe involves preparing a cucumber and mint smoothie. First, peel and slice a cucumber and remove the mint leaves. Blend the ingredients in a blender, adding plain yogurt and water. Optionally, add a teaspoon of honey for sweetness. Blend until smooth, creating a refreshing green smoothie. Taste and adjust the sweetness to your desired level. Add more honey or water if needed. Serve and chill the smoothie in a glass, garnished with fresh mint. Adjust the smoothie's thickness by adding more or less water. For added health benefits, consider using Greek yogurt, which is higher in protein and can make the smoothie creamier. For a cooler taste, use chilled cucumber and yogurt or add ice cubes when blending.

3. Spinach and Banana Delight

Ingredients:

- 1 cup of fresh spinach
- 1 ripe banana
- 1/2 cup of unsweetened almond milk
- 1 tablespoon of flaxseed meal

Instructions:

Ripe bananas and fresh spinach must be prepared for this recipe. The banana is sliced into smaller pieces, and the spinach is cleaned. Using a blender, combine the ingredients until they have a smooth, creamy texture. The natural sweetness of the banana combines with the vivid green hue of the spinach. You may change the smoothie's consistency by adding more almond milk. After that, the smoothie is served in a glass with ripe banana added for sweetness and flaxseed meal for texture and nutritional value. Protein powder may be added to the smoothie to give it an additional boost. This smoothie is tasty and easy to make, making it a great choice for a nutritious breakfast.

4. Apple Pie Smoothie

Ingredients:

- 1 apple, peeled, cored, and chopped
- 1/2 teaspoon of ground cinnamon
- 1/2 cup of plain yogurt
- 1/2 cup of water
- 1 tablespoon of honey (optional)

Instructions:

Peel, core, and cut 1 apple (ideally a sweet type like Fuji or Honeycrisp) to make a smoothie for this recipe. After blending the ingredients, a spoonful of honey is added for sweetness. After that, the smoothie is mixed until it is creamy and smooth, tasting like an apple pie. You may change the consistency by adding more water, and you can alter the sweetness by adding more honey or water. Serve the Apple Pie Smoothie in a glass, top with some cinnamon, and pair it with some warm apple pie. Ripe apples are used in this recipe to give it a naturally sweet flavor, and you may change the amount of cinnamon to your own taste. While mixing, you may add cold apple slices and yogurt or ice cubes to make the smoothie more refreshing.

5. Tropical Twist

Ingredients:

- 1/2 cup of pineapple chunks
- 1/2 cup of mango chunks
- 1/2 cup of coconut milk
- 1/2 cup of water
- 1 tablespoon of honey (optional)

Instructions:

To make a Tropical Twist Smoothie, combine pineapple and mango chunks, coconut milk, and water in a blender. Optionally, add a tablespoon of honey for a sweeter taste. Blend until smooth and creamy, capturing the essence of a tropical paradise. Taste the smoothie to adjust sweetness and consistency by adding more honey or water. Serve and enjoy the exotic and kidney-friendly flavors by pouring it into a glass, garnishing with a slice of pineapple or mango, and enjoying the exotic and kidney-friendly flavors. If fresh fruit is unavailable, use canned pineapple and mango chunks in juice or water, draining them before blending. For extra frostiness, use frozen fruit or ice cubes while blending. For a zesty twist, add a dash of lime or lemon juice for a refreshing tang to the tropical flavors.

6. Avocado Banana Smoothie

Ingredients:

- 1/2 ripe avocado
- 1 ripe banana
- 1/2 cup of unsweetened almond milk
- 1 tablespoon of honey (optional)

Instructions:

In order to make this recipe, ripe avocados and bananas are blended into a creamy smoothie. Add the avocado, banana, unsweetened almond milk, and optional honey to the smoothie. Let the natural creaminess of the avocado come through by blending until smooth and creamy. Taste the smoothie and add additional honey or almond milk to suit your desired consistency and sweetness levels. Garnish the smoothie with avocado or banana slices after serving it in a glass, then savor its rich, kidney-friendly flavors. Use a ripe banana with brown speckles to intensify the sweetness so that it tastes good without the need for additional sweeteners. You can use it if you'd rather use almond, soy, or coconut milk, for example. When blending, add ice cubes or use frozen banana slices to make the smoothie extra cold.

7. Carrot Cake Smoothie

Ingredients:

- 1 small carrot, peeled and chopped
- 1/2 cup of plain yogurt
- 1/2 cup of unsweetened almond milk
- 1/4 cup of rolled oats
- 1/2 teaspoon of ground cinnamon
- 1/4 teaspoon of ground nutmeg
- 1/4 teaspoon of vanilla extract
- 1 tablespoon of honey (optional)

Instructions:

Peel and cut a small carrot into tiny pieces for easy blending while making a Carrot Cake Smoothie. In a blender, combine the carrot, plain yogurt, honey, unsweetened almond milk, rolled oats, ground nutmeg, ground cinnamon, and vanilla extract until smooth and creamy. For sweetness, you can optionally add one tablespoon of honey. Blend till consistency of cake is reached. After tasting the smoothie, add extra honey, almond milk, or spices to suit your preference for sweetness, thickness, or spice levels. Pour the Carrot Cake Smoothie into a glass, top with shredded carrot or cinnamon, and savor the flavors that are good for your kidneys and cozy. Use a small sweet carrot for a naturally sweet flavor. You may also use less liquid for a thicker consistency or change the thickness by adding more or less almond milk. When combining, add ice cubes for additional cooling.

8. Peachy Green Smoothie

Ingredients:

- 1 peach, peeled and pitted
- 1 cup of fresh spinach
- 1/2 cup of plain yogurt
- 1/2 cup of water
- 1 tablespoon of honey (optional)

Instructions:

This recipe involves preparing a peach smoothie by peeling and pitting it, blending it with spinach, yogurt, and water, and adding honey for sweetness. The smoothie can be adjusted by adding more honey or water to suit your taste. Once blended, it should be served in a glass, garnished with a slice of peach or spinach leaves, and enjoyed with a refreshing and kidney-friendly flavor. To ensure the smoothie is as sweet as desired, use a ripe peach that yields slightly when gently pressed. Adjust the smoothie's thickness by adding more or less water, depending on your preference. For an extra chill, use chilled peach and yogurt or add ice cubes while blending. The recipe is simple and delicious, making it a great way to enjoy a refreshing and kidney-friendly beverage.

9. Cherry Almond Delight

Ingredients:

- 1/2 cup of pitted cherries (fresh or frozen)
- 1/4 cup of unsalted almonds
- 1/2 cup of almond milk
- 1/2 cup of water
- 1 tablespoon of honey (optional)

Instructions:

This recipe involves blending cherries, unsalted almonds, almond milk, and water in a blender. If using fresh cherries, remove the pits and thaw them before blending. If using frozen cherries, thaw them before blending. If adding honey, add a tablespoon for sweetness. Blend until smooth and luscious, then taste and adjust the sweetness, thickness, or consistency by adding more honey or water. Serve and enjoy the Cherry Almond Delight Smoothie in a glass, garnished with cherries or crushed almonds for elegance. Tip: Use fresh or frozen cherries depending on availability and preference. For extra almond flavor, add a drop of almond extract, but use it sparingly due to its strong taste. For a frosty sensation, use frozen cherries or ice cubes while blending.

10. Pomegranate Berry Smoothie

Ingredients:

- 1/2 cup of pomegranate seeds or 100% pomegranate juice
- 1/2 cup of mixed berries (blueberries, strawberries, raspberries)
- 1/2 cup of plain yogurt
- 1/2 cup of water
- 1 tablespoon of honey (optional)

Instructions:

This recipe involves preparing pomegranate seeds or juice, blending the antioxidant mix, adding honey, and blending until a berry smoothie. The ingredients are mixed together until smooth and luscious, capturing the flavors of pomegranate and berries. The sweetness can be adjusted by adding more honey or water to taste. The smoothie can be served in a glass, garnished with mixed berries for an elegant touch, and savor the antioxidant-rich and kidney-friendly flavors. To save time, pre-packaged pomegranate seeds can be purchased in grocery stores. Mixed berries can be fresh or frozen, and frozen berries or ice cubes can be added for a refreshing twist. The recipe is suitable for those who prefer a more sweet taste.

11. Almond Butter Banana Smoothie

Ingredients:

- 1 ripe banana
- 2 tablespoons of almond butter
- 1/2 cup of plain yogurt
- 1/2 cup of almond milk
- 1 tablespoon of honey (optional)

Instructions:

This recipe involves preparing a banana smoothie by peeling and breaking it into smaller chunks. The smoothie is then blended with banana chunks, almond butter, plain yogurt, almond milk, and honey. If desired, honey can be added for sweetness. The mixture is then blended until a nutty blend is achieved. The sweetness can be adjusted by adding more honey or almond milk to taste. The smoothie can be served in a glass, garnished with almond butter or a slice of banana, and enjoyed with a drizzle of almond butter or a slice of banana. For a creamier texture and extra protein, Greek yogurt can be used instead of plain yogurt. The thickness can be customized by adding more or less almond milk, and a frostier experience can be achieved by using chilled banana and almond milk or adding ice cubes while blending.

12. Spinach and Pineapple Green Smoothie

Ingredients:

- 1 cup of fresh spinach
- 1/2 cup of pineapple chunks (fresh or frozen)
- 1/2 cup of plain yogurt
- 1/2 cup of water
- 1 tablespoon of honey (optional)

Instructions:

This recipe calls for combining water, plain yogurt, pineapple chunks, and fresh spinach to make a cool, tropical smoothie. One tablespoon of honey can be added for sweetness, or left out if preferred. Blend till smooth and energizing, retaining the nutritious value of spinach and the tropical aroma of pineapple. Add more honey or water based on your taste to change the smoothie's sweetness, thickness, or consistency. Pour the smoothie into a glass, top with some fresh spinach leaves or a pineapple slice, and savor the flavors—which are good for your kidneys and energizing. Use frozen pineapple chunks, Greek yogurt, or ice cubes when mixing for a refreshing experience. Add more or less water to adjust the smoothie's thickness. For a zesty touch, consider adding a dash of lemon or lime juice.

13. Oatmeal Cookie Smoothie

Ingredients:

- 1/2 cup of rolled oats
- 1 ripe banana
- 1/2 teaspoon of ground cinnamon
- 1/4 teaspoon of ground nutmeg
- 1/2 cup of plain yogurt
- 1/2 cup of water

- 1 tablespoon of honey (optional)

Instructions:

To make an oatmeal cookie smoothie, blend rolled oats, ripe banana, ground cinnamon, ground nutmeg, plain yogurt, and water until fine. Optionally, add a tablespoon of honey for a sweeter taste. Blend until a smooth, creamy consistency resembles an oatmeal cookie. Taste the smoothie to adjust sweetness, thickness, or consistency by adding more honey or water. Serve and enjoy the comforting and kidney-friendly flavors by pouring it into a glass, garnishing with cinnamon or ground nutmeg. For natural sweetness, use a ripe banana with brown speckles. Adjust the smoothie's thickness by adding more or less water, depending on your preference. For an extra chill, use chilled banana, yogurt, or ice cubes while blending.

14. Watermelon Mint Cooler

Ingredients:

- 1 1/2 cups of fresh watermelon, diced and seedless
- 6-8 fresh mint leaves
- 1/2 cup of plain yogurt
- 1/4 cup of water
- 1 tablespoon of honey (optional)

Instructions:

This recipe turns plain yogurt, water, mint leaves, and sliced fresh watermelon into a cool smoothie. For sweetness, you can optionally add honey, but taste first. Process till minty and smooth, retaining the refreshing flavor of watermelon and mint. Taste and add extra honey or water to suit your taste in order to change sweetness, thickness, or consistency. Garnish the cool smoothie with slices of watermelon or fresh mint and serve. Use cold watermelon chunks, yogurt, or ice cubes in the blender for an additional chilly experience. Depending on your choice, you may add more or less water to change the smoothie's thickness. Add a squeeze of fresh lemon or lime juice for a zesty flavor.

15. Raspberry Almond Protein Smoothie

Ingredients:

- 1/2 cup of frozen raspberries
- 1/4 cup of unsalted almonds
- 1/2 cup of plain yogurt
- 1/2 cup of almond milk
- 1 tablespoon of honey (optional)

- 1 scoop of your favorite vanilla or unflavored protein powder (optional)

Instructions:

To make a refreshing Raspberry Almond Protein Smoothie, freeze fresh raspberries in advance. Blend plain yogurt, almond milk, frozen raspberries, unsalted almonds, and honey in a blender until smooth and creamy. Optionally, add protein powder to increase protein content. Taste the smoothie's sweetness and adjust with honey or almond milk to change sweetness, thickness, or consistency. Serve the smoothie in a glass with raspberries or crushed almonds for a decorative touch. For a colder experience, use frozen raspberries or ice cubes in the blender. Almond extract should be used sparingly to accentuate the nutty flavor. If taking a protein supplement, ensure it fits within your diet and is kidney-friendly.

16. Blueberry Spinach Smoothie

Ingredients:

- 1/2 cup of fresh or frozen blueberries
- 1 cup of fresh spinach
- 1/2 cup of plain yogurt
- 1/2 cup of water

- 1 tablespoon of honey (optional)

Instructions:

This recipe involves preparing blueberries, spinach, water, plain yogurt, and honey in a blender. The blueberries should be rinsed and frozen if used. The smoothie should be blended until smooth and vibrant, combining the flavors of blueberries and spinach. If needed, honey can be added for sweetness. The smoothie should be tasted and adjusted to achieve the desired consistency. The smoothie can be served in a glass with fresh blueberries or spinach leaves for a visually appealing presentation. For a refreshing experience, use cold blueberries or yogurt or add ice cubes to the blender. For added fiber and omega-3 fatty acids, add a tablespoon of flaxseed meal or chia seeds. The consistency can be adjusted by adding more water or yogurt. The recipe is recommended for those looking for a healthy and antioxidant-rich smoothie.

17. Carrot Ginger Delight

Ingredients:

- 1 large carrot, peeled and chopped
- 1/2 inch piece of fresh ginger, peeled

- 1/2 cup of plain yogurt
- 1/2 cup of water
- 1 tablespoon of honey (optional)

Instructions:

To make the Carrot Ginger Delight Smoothie, peel and cut a giant carrot into smaller pieces and slice the raw ginger thinly. In a blender, combine water, plain yogurt, sliced carrot, and fresh ginger slices. Optionally, add honey for sweetness. Blend until a creamy, tangy smoothie combines the subtle sweetness of carrots with the strong flavor of ginger. Taste and adjust the smoothie's sweetness with a spoonful of honey. Add additional water or honey to adjust the consistency. Transfer the smoothie into a glass, add a carrot twist or slice of fresh ginger for visual appeal, and enjoy the kidney-friendly and revitalizing taste. For a more subdued ginger taste, use a smaller piece of fresh ginger. Use cold carrot slices or yogurt or combine in ice cubes for a refreshing experience. Personalize the smoothie by adding ground cinnamon or fresh lime juice. This zesty and delicious approach to kidney function promotes kidney function, especially after a transplant.

18. Mango Banana Coconut Smoothie

Ingredients:

- 1/2 cup of fresh or frozen mango chunks
- 1 ripe banana
- 1/2 cup of unsweetened coconut milk
- 1/2 cup of plain yogurt
- 1 tablespoon of honey (optional)

Instructions:

This recipe for a tropical smoothie involves blending mango chunks, ripe banana pieces, plain yogurt, unsweetened coconut milk, and honey in a blender. If using frozen mango, allow it to defrost before mixing. If using fresh mango, peel it and cut it into smaller pieces. The smoothie is then blended until a smooth, tropical smoothie is formed, encapsulating the unique tastes of coconut and mango. The sweetness can be adjusted by adding honey or coconut milk to suit the taste. The smoothie can be served in a glass, topped with a mango slice or shredded coconut for a unique look. For an additional tropical taste, try using coconut yogurt instead of plain yogurt, adding ice cubes or frozen mango chunks while mixing, or adding a squeeze of fresh lime juice for a tangy kick. This smoothie promotes kidney function, especially after a transplant, by fusing the creaminess of coconut with the pleasant sweetness of mango.

19. Blackberry Walnut Bliss

Ingredients:

- 1/2 cup of fresh blackberries
- 1/4 cup of unsalted walnuts
- 1/2 cup of plain yogurt
- 1/2 cup of water
- 1 tablespoon of honey (optional)

Instructions:

This recipe for a Blackberry Walnut Bliss Smoothie is a delicious and nutritious way to maintain kidney function, especially after a transplant. To make the smoothie, rinse fresh blackberries and combine water, plain yogurt, blackberries, and unsalted walnuts in a blender. Optionally, add honey for sweetness. Blend until a smooth, nutty mixture forms, combining the rich walnut tastes and tart blackberry notes. Taste the smoothie and adjust the sweetness with water or honey to achieve the desired consistency. Serve the smoothie in a glass with a blackberry or walnut half as a garnish. For a chilly and refreshing taste, use frozen blackberries or yogurt, or add ice cubes to the blender. Personalize the smoothie with cinnamon for a touch of spice. Greek yogurt may give the dish a creamier texture. Overall, this smoothie is a delicious and nutritious way to enjoy the rich, nutty taste of blackberries and walnuts.

20. Strawberry Cucumber Refresher

Ingredients:

- 1 cup of fresh strawberries, hulled and halved
- 1/2 cup of fresh cucumber, peeled and sliced
- 1/2 cup of plain yogurt
- 1/2 cup of water
- 1 tablespoon of honey (optional)

Instructions:

To make a Strawberry Cucumber Refresher Smoothie, cut fresh strawberries and cucumbers into half and peel them. In a blender, combine water, plain yogurt, cucumber slices, and halved strawberries. Optionally, add honey for sweetness. Blend until a refreshing blend, combining cucumber's sharpness with strawberries' juiciness. Taste and adjust sweetness as needed. Add more water or honey to achieve the desired consistency. Serve in a glass with a slice of cucumber or a strawberry for a cool touch. For a chilly taste, use cold strawberries or yogurt, or add ice cubes to the blender. For citrus, add fresh lime or lemon juice.

For herbal freshness, add mint leaves. This refreshing and cold smoothie is a great way to maintain kidney function, especially after a transplant, and enjoy the sweet, juicy strawberries and crisp cucumbers. It tastes refreshing and cold like a summer sip.

21. Papaya Passion Smoothie

Ingredients:

- 1/2 cup of fresh papaya, cubed
- 1 passion fruit, pulp and seeds
- 1/2 cup of plain yogurt
- 1/2 cup of water
- 1 tablespoon of honey (optional)

Instructions:

The Papaya Passion Smoothie is a tropical drink that promotes kidney health, especially after a transplant, by combining the distinct taste of passion fruit with the delicious sweetness of papaya. To make it, gather the pulp and seeds from the passion fruit, cube the fresh papaya, and combine the ingredients in a blender. Optionally, add honey for sweetness, but adjust the sweetness after tasting. Blend until a smooth, tropical concoction forms, encapsulating the unique tastes of passion fruit and papaya. Taste and adjust the smoothie's sweetness to get the desired consistency. Serve and enjoy the tropical taste in a glass, adding a piece of papaya or passion fruit for an exotic touch. For a refreshing twist, add ice cubes, chilled papaya or yogurt cubes, coconut milk, or fresh lime or lemon juice. This tropical paradise is similar to enjoying a tropical beverage at home.

22. Banana Walnut Breakfast Smoothie

Ingredients:

- 1 ripe banana
- 1/4 cup of unsalted walnuts
- 1/2 cup of rolled oats
- 1/2 cup of plain yogurt
- 1/2 cup of milk (dairy or plant-based)
- 1 tablespoon of honey (optional)

Instructions:

This recipe for a Banana Walnut Breakfast Smoothie is a simple and nutritious way to start the day. To make it, cut ripe bananas into smaller pieces and blend the hearty mixture with milk, plain yogurt, rolled oats, and unsalted walnuts. Optionally, add honey for sweetness. Blend until a smooth, nutty, and hearty consistency is achieved, combining the crunch of walnuts with the sweetness of the bananas. Taste and adjust the sweetness as needed. Serve the smoothie in a glass, top with a slice of banana or chopped walnuts for a hearty touch, and enjoy the nutty, stimulating, and kidney-healthy taste. For a cooler smoothie, use a frozen banana or ice cubes while mixing. Experiment with adding nutmeg or cinnamon for additional flavor. Greek yogurt may provide more creaminess and protein than plain yogurt. This nutritious and filling breakfast choice enhances kidney function, especially after a transplant, by blending the natural sweetness of bananas with the crunch of walnuts.

23. Kiwi Lime Cooler

Ingredients:

- 2 ripe kiwis, peeled and sliced
- Juice of 1 fresh lime
- 1/2 cup of plain yogurt
- 1/2 cup of water
- 1 tablespoon of honey (optional)

Instructions:

The Kiwi Lime Cooler Smoothie is a refreshing and zesty way to maintain kidney function, especially after kidney transplant surgery. To make it, cut and peel ripe kiwis and extract the juice of a fresh lime. Blend the water, plain yogurt, and kiwis in a blender until a zesty blend is formed. If desired, add honey for sweetness. Taste the smoothie and adjust the sweetness, thickness, or consistency as needed. Pour the smoothie into a glass, add a lime wheel or kiwi slice for a zesty touch, and enjoy the gentle kidney-friendly taste. For a more refreshing experience, mix ice cubes or use cooled yogurt or kiwi slices. Add fresh mint leaves for a herbal edge to the spicy taste or lime zest for a citrus punch. The Kiwi Lime Cooler Smoothie is a refreshing and refreshing way to maintain kidney function, making it a great choice for those after kidney transplant surgery.

24. High-Protein Smoothie with Peaches

Ingredients:

- 1 ripe peach, pitted and chopped
- 1/2 cup of Greek yogurt
- 1/2 cup of cottage cheese
- 1/2 cup of almond milk (or any milk of your choice)
- 1 scoop of vanilla protein powder
- 1 tablespoon of honey (optional, for added sweetness)

Instructions:

This recipe involves preparing a high-protein peach smoothie by combining ripe peaches, Greek yogurt, cottage cheese, almond milk, protein powder, vanilla extract, and honey. Optional honey can be added for sweetness, but taste is crucial. Blend the ingredients until smooth and creamy, fusing protein-rich components with peach flavors. Taste and adjust sweetness as needed. Transfer the smoothie to a glass, add a peach slice or honey drizzle for visual appeal, and enjoy the rich, creamy, and peach flavors. For a creamier and cooler experience, use frozen peach slices or ice cubes. For added nutrients and fiber, consider adding chia seeds or spinach. Tailor the protein powder to your taste and brand. This smoothie is a great option for those trying to consume more protein while enjoying the delicious taste of peaches.

25. Vanilla Almond Smoothie

Ingredients:

- 1 cup of almond milk
- 1 ripe banana
- 1/4 cup of unsalted almonds
- 1 teaspoon of pure vanilla extract

- 1 tablespoon of honey (optional, for added sweetness)

Instructions:

This recipe involves preparing a Vanilla Almond Smoothie by cutting a ripe banana into pieces and blending the almond milk, ripe banana, almonds, pure vanilla essence, and honey. If desired, honey can be added for sweetness. The smoothie is then blended until a smooth and creamy texture is achieved, blending the almond nuttiness with the soothing vanilla taste. The sweetness can be adjusted by adding more honey or almond milk to suit the taste. The smoothie can be served and enjoyed by adding a banana slice or chopped almonds as a garnish. For a more refreshing experience, use cold almond milk or pulse in ice cubes. For a touch of spice, add a dash of ground cinnamon. For a thicker consistency, add rolled oats or additional almonds. The Vanilla Almond Smoothie is a creamy and delectable combination of vanilla and almond goodness, making it a tasty and healthy addition to your smoothie routine.

26. Blueberry Oatmeal Smoothie

Ingredients:

- 1/2 cup of fresh or frozen blueberries
- 1/2 cup of rolled oats
- 1/2 cup of plain yogurt
- 1/2 cup of almond milk (or any milk of your choice)
- 1 tablespoon of honey (optional, for added sweetness)

Instructions:

This recipe involves preparing blueberries, rolled oats, plain yogurt, almond milk, and honey in a blender. If using fresh blueberries, rinse them and if using the frozen ones, let them defrost slightly. In a blender, combine the nutrient-rich mixture, optionally adding honey for sweetness. Blend until a creamy, nutrient-dense mix forms, combining the antioxidant-rich taste of blueberries with the filling strength of oats. Taste and adjust the sweetness to get the desired consistency. Adjust the sweetness, thickness, or consistency as needed. Serve the smoothie in a glass, top with blueberries or oats for a healthy twist. For a creamier and cooler experience, use frozen blueberries or ice cubes. Add almond butter or cinnamon for flavor or use a ripe banana or sweetened yogurt instead of honey. This smoothie is a satisfying and healthy way to enjoy the satisfying combination of oats and blueberry antioxidants.

27. Cherry Coconut Dream

Ingredients:

- 1/2 cup of fresh or frozen cherries, pitted
- 1/2 cup of coconut milk
- 1/2 cup of plain yogurt
- 1 tablespoon of honey (optional, for added sweetness)

Instructions:

The Cherry Coconut Dream Smoothie is a tropical blend of sweet-tart cherries and exotic coconut, perfect for a tropical paradise in a glass. To prepare, remove the pits from fresh cherries and let them defrost slightly. Blend the ingredients in a blender, adding honey if needed. Blend until the mixture combines the sweet-tart tastes of cherries with the exotic deliciousness of coconut, creating a creamy and dreamy consistency. Taste and adjust the sweetness to suit your taste. Serve the smoothie with a cherry or shredded coconut for a touch of the tropics. For a refreshing experience, use frozen cherries or coconut milk, or combine in ice cubes. For a zesty touch, add a squeeze of fresh lime juice. For a stronger coconut taste, try using coconut yogurt. This refreshing and kidney-friendly smoothie is similar to enjoying a tropical beverage at home.

28. Mango Spinach Green Smoothie

Ingredients:

- 1/2 cup of fresh or frozen mango chunks
- 1 cup of fresh spinach leaves
- 1/2 cup of plain yogurt
- 1/2 cup of water
- 1 tablespoon of honey (optional, for added sweetness)

Instructions:

This recipe for a mango spinach green smoothie involves preparing ingredients such as fresh mango, spinach leaves, water, plain yogurt, and honey. The smoothie is then blended until a smooth and refreshing consistency is reached, combining the nutritional properties of spinach with the tropical sweetness of mango. The smoothie's sweetness can be adjusted by adding more water or honey, or by adjusting the sweetness, thickness, or consistency. The smoothie can be served in a glass, topped with spinach leaves or a slice of mango for a cool touch. For a more refreshing taste, frozen mango chunks or yogurt can be added, or ice cubes can be added. A squeeze of fresh lime or lemon juice can also be added for a zesty touch. Chia seeds can be added to increase fiber and omega-3 fatty acids. This nutrient-rich, refreshing drink boosts kidney health by combining the tropical taste of mango with the leafy benefits of spinach.

29. Raspberry Peach Bliss

Ingredients:

- 1/2 cup of fresh or frozen raspberries
- 1 ripe peach, pitted and sliced
- 1/2 cup of plain yogurt
- 1/2 cup of water
- 1 tablespoon of honey (optional, for added sweetness)

Instructions:

This recipe involves preparing raspberries, ripe peaches, water, plain yogurt, and honey in a blender. The mixture should be a smooth, sweet-tart consistency, blending the flavors of raspberries and peaches. If desired, honey can be added for sweetness. The smoothie should be tasted and adjusted to achieve the desired consistency. The final product should be served in a glass with a slice of peach or raspberry for visual appeal. For a refreshing experience, use cold yogurt or raspberries, or combine with ice cubes. For a zesty touch, add a squeeze of fresh lime or lemon juice. Ground flaxseeds can be added to increase fiber and omega-3 fatty acids. This recipe offers a fruity pleasure experience, promoting kidney health while enjoying the tropical sweetness of peaches and the sweet-tartness of raspberries.

30. Lemon Berry Zest

Ingredients:

- 1 cup of mixed berries (strawberries, blueberries, raspberries, blackberries)
- Juice of 1 lemon
- 1/2 cup of plain yogurt
- 1/2 cup of water
- 1 tablespoon of honey (optional, for added sweetness)

Instructions:

This recipe involves blending mixed berries and lemon juice in a blender, combining water, plain yogurt, lemon juice, and mixed berries. Optional honey can be added for sweetness, but taste is crucial. Blend until the mixture combines the sweet burst of mixed berries with the tang of lemon, creating a smooth and zesty consistency. Adjust the sweetness by adding more water or honey, or adjusting the thickness or consistency. Serve the smoothie in a glass with a mixed berry or lemon wheel as a zesty garnish. For a refreshing taste, use cooled mixed berries or yogurt, or add ice cubes to the blender. For a revitalizing herbal touch, add mint leaves or chia seeds. This kidney-friendly smoothie is a delicious and zesty way to enjoy the sweet sweetness of mixed berries with the zing of lemon. It tastes like a sip of sunlight in a glass.

31. Green Apple Cinnamon Smoothie

Ingredients:

- 1 green apple, cored and sliced
- 1/2 teaspoon of ground cinnamon
- 1/2 cup of plain yogurt
- 1/2 cup of water
- 1 tablespoon of honey (optional, for added sweetness)

Instructions:

This recipe involves blending a green apple cinnamon smoothie with plain yogurt, water, ground cinnamon, and green apple slices. Optional honey can be added for sweetness, but taste is crucial. Blend until a refreshing and aromatic consistency is achieved, blending the cinnamon's warmth with the crispness of the green apples. Adjust sweetness as needed, adding more water or honey if needed. Serve in a glass with a piece of green apple or cinnamon dusting for visual appeal. For a refreshing experience, use cold green apple slices or yogurt, or add ice cubes to the blender. For added nutrition, add spinach leaves or Greek yogurt for more protein and a creamier texture. Enjoy the light, fragrant, and kidney-healthy flavors.

32. Banana Blueberry Chia Smoothie

Ingredients:

- 1 ripe banana
- 1/2 cup of blueberries (fresh or frozen)
- 1 tablespoon of chia seeds
- 1/2 cup of plain yogurt
- 1/2 cup of water
- 1 tablespoon of honey (optional, for added sweetness)

Instructions:

This recipe for a Banana Blueberry Chia Smoothie involves preparing ingredients such as ripe banana, rinsed blueberries, plain yogurt, honey, and chia seeds. Blend the smoothie until it reaches a creamy and nutrient-rich consistency. The smoothie is made by combining antioxidant-rich blueberries, naturally sweet bananas, and the nutritional benefits of chia seeds. The sweetness can be adjusted by adding more water or honey, or by adjusting the sweetness, thickness, or consistency. The smoothie can be served in a glass with a blueberry or chia seed for a visually pleasing touch. For a refreshing experience, use cold blueberries or yogurt or add ice cubes to the blender. For additional flavor, try vanilla extract or cinnamon. Chia seeds absorb moisture and add thickness, so adjust the water quantity accordingly.

33. Spinach and Pineapple Protein Boost

Ingredients:

- 1 cup of fresh spinach leaves
- 1/2 cup of pineapple chunks (fresh or frozen)
- 1/2 cup of Greek yogurt
- 1/2 cup of water
- 1 scoop of vanilla protein powder
- 1 tablespoon of honey (optional, for added sweetness)

Instructions:

This recipe involves preparing fresh spinach leaves and chopping pineapple into bits. The ingredients are then combined in a blender with Greek yogurt, spinach leaves, water, vanilla protein powder, and honey. If desired, honey can be added for sweetness. Blend the smoothie in a blender until a smooth, nutrient-rich consistency is achieved. The sweetness can be adjusted by adding more water or honey, or by adjusting the thickness or consistency. The smoothie is served in a glass, topped with a fresh pineapple slice or spinach leaf for a visually pleasing finish. For a refreshing experience, use cold pineapple chunks or yogurt or ice cubes. For a zesty twist, add a squeeze of fresh lime or lemon juice. The protein powder should be tailored to your desired taste and brand, ensuring it meets your nutritional requirements.

34. Carrot-Orange Sunshine Smoothie

Ingredients:

- 2 large carrots, peeled and chopped
- Juice of 2 oranges
- 1/2 cup of plain yogurt
- 1/2 cup of water
- 1 tablespoon of honey (optional, for added sweetness)

Instructions:

This recipe involves preparing carrots and oranges, blending them into a Sunshine Mixture. The ingredients include chopped carrots, water, orange juice, plain yogurt, and honey. If desired, honey can be added for sweetness. Blend until a smooth and nourishing consistency is achieved, blending the earthy richness of carrots with the natural sweetness of oranges. Taste the smoothie and adjust the sweetness, thickness, or consistency as needed. Serve the Carrot-Orange Sunshine Smoothie in a glass with a carrot ribbon or slice of orange for a colorful touch. For a refreshing taste, use cold orange juice or yogurt, or add ice cubes to the blender. For a spicy kick, sprinkle ground ginger and a teaspoon of turmeric for antioxidants. This recipe is kidney-friendly, nourishing.

35. Simple Protein Smoothie with Pineapple

Ingredients:

- 1 cup of pineapple chunks (fresh or frozen)
- 1/2 cup of Greek yogurt
- 1/2 cup of water
- 1 scoop of your preferred protein powder (vanilla or unflavored)

- 1 tablespoon of honey (optional, for added sweetness)

Instructions:

This recipe involves preparing a Pineapple Simple Protein Smoothie by combining Greek yogurt, pineapple chunks, water, protein powder, and honey in a blender. Optional honey can be added for sweetness, but taste is crucial. Blend until a smooth and protein-rich consistency is achieved, blending the protein-rich powder with the tropical sweetness of the pineapple. Taste and adjust the consistency as needed, adding more water or honey if needed. Serve the smoothie in a glass with a pineapple chunk or honey drizzle for visual appeal. For a refreshing experience, use cold pineapple chunks or yogurt or ice cubes. For added flavor, add a pinch of cinnamon. Tailor the protein powder to your taste and brand, ensuring it meets your nutritional requirements.

36. Smoothie with Fruit

Ingredients:

- 1/2 cup of strawberries (fresh or frozen)
- 1/2 cup of blueberries (fresh or frozen)
- 1/2 cup of chopped mango (fresh or frozen)

- 1/2 banana
- 1/2 cup of plain yogurt
- 1/2 cup of orange juice
- 1 tablespoon of honey (optional, for added sweetness)

Instructions:

This recipe involves preparing ingredients such as strawberries, blueberries, mango, and banana. In a blender, blend orange juice, plain yogurt, banana, sliced mango, blueberries, and strawberries. Optionally, add honey for sweetness. Mix until smooth and delicious, then taste and adjust sweetness as needed. Add additional honey or orange juice to change sweetness, thickness, or consistency. Serve and enjoy the mixed fruit smoothie in a glass with a fruit slice or honey drizzle for visual appeal. For a refreshing experience, use cold fruit or yogurt or combine with ice cubes. For added nutrients, add kale or spinach, and for fiber and omega-3 fatty acids, add chia or flax seeds. The smoothie is kidney-friendly, creamy, and mixed fruit-based.

37. Protein Shake with Mixed Berries

Ingredients:

- 1/2 cup of mixed berries (strawberries, blueberries, raspberries, blackberries)
- 1/2 cup of Greek yogurt
- 1/2 cup of water
- 1 scoop of your preferred protein powder (vanilla or unflavored)
- 1 tablespoon of honey (optional, for added sweetness)

Instructions:

This protein shake with mixed berries is a delicious and nutrient-rich option for a high-protein snack or lunch substitute. To make it, rinse fresh and frozen berries, blend Greek yogurt, mixed berries, water, protein powder, and honey in a blender. Optionally, add honey for sweetness, but taste the shake to determine if more is needed. Blend until a creamy and protein-rich consistency is achieved, combining the protein-boosting power of the powder with the antioxidant-dense tastes of mixed berries. Adjust the sweetness level with a taste, adding more water or honey, or adjusting the consistency. Serve and enjoy the delicious taste of this protein shake, rich in protein, fruit, and good for kidney health. For a refreshing experience, use cold yogurt or berries, or combine with ice cubes. Add spinach or kale for more nutrients, or chia or flax seeds for fiber and omega-3 fatty acids. This high-protein snack or lunch substitute is a satisfying and kidney-friendly option for a satisfying and nutritious meal.

38. Pineapple Mint Refresher

Ingredients:

- 1 cup of fresh pineapple chunks
- 5-6 fresh mint leaves
- 1/2 cup of water
- 1/2 cup of ice cubes
- 1 tablespoon of honey (optional, for added sweetness)

Instructions:

To make a refreshing Pineapple Mint Refresher, chop fresh pineapple and rinse mint leaves. Blend pineapple chunks, water, ice cubes, mint leaves, and honey in a blender. Optionally, add honey for sweetness. Blend until a cold, refreshing texture is achieved, blending the sweet tang of pineapple with the energizing flavor of mint. Taste and adjust the sweetness by adding more water or honey, or adjusting sweetness, thickness, or consistency. Serve the refreshing Pineapple Mint Refresher in a glass, top with a piece of pineapple or mint leaf for a nice touch, and enjoy the cool, tropical, and kidney-friendly taste. For a more refreshing and chilly experience, add more ice cubes or use cooled pineapple or mint leaves. For a zesty touch, add a splash of fresh lime juice. For a contrast of sweet and salty, add a teaspoon of salt. This refreshing and kidney-friendly recipe offers a taste of the tropics at home.

39. High-Protein Strawberry Smoothie

Ingredients:

- 1 cup of fresh strawberries
- 1/2 cup of Greek yogurt
- 1/2 cup of milk (dairy or non-dairy)
- 1/2 cup of rolled oats
- 1 scoop of your preferred protein powder (vanilla or strawberry flavor)
- 1 tablespoon of honey (optional, for added sweetness)

Instructions:

This recipe for a High-Protein Strawberry Smoothie involves preparing fresh strawberries, blending them with Greek yogurt, milk, rolled oats, protein powder, and honey. Optional honey can be added for sweetness. The smoothie is then mixed until smooth and protein-rich, combining the Greek yogurt and protein powder with the naturally sweet strawberries. Taste and adjust the sweetness to get the desired consistency. Pour the smoothie into a glass, top with honey or fresh strawberries, and enjoy the rich protein, fruit, and kidney-friendly taste. For a refreshing taste, use cold strawberries or yogurt, or add ice cubes to the blender. For added nutrition, add baby spinach for added nutrition. Tailor the protein powder to your desired taste and brand. This delicious and kidney-friendly option is perfect for refueling after a workout or for breakfast.

40. Mixed Berry Spinach Delight

Ingredients:

- 1/2 cup of mixed berries (strawberries, blueberries, raspberries, blackberries)
- 1 cup of fresh spinach leaves
- 1/2 cup of plain yogurt
- 1/2 cup of water
- 1 tablespoon of honey (optional, for added sweetness)

Instructions:

This recipe for a Mixed Berry Spinach Delight Smoothie is a nutritious and delicious way to enjoy a healthy breakfast or snack. To make it, rinse fresh berries and thoroughly wash raw spinach leaves. Blend the mixed berries, water, plain yogurt, and spinach leaves in a blender until a smooth and nutrient-rich consistency is achieved. If desired, add honey for sweetness. Taste the smoothie and adjust the sweetness, thickness, or consistency as needed. Serve the smoothie in a glass with a mixed berry or spinach leaf for visual appeal. For a refreshing experience, use cold yogurt or berries, or combine with ice cubes. For a zesty twist, add lemon juice. For increased fiber and omega-3 fatty acids, add one tablespoon of ground flaxseeds. This nutritious and delicious kidney-friendly smoothie is a great option for a healthy breakfast or snack.

CONCLUSION

"The Ultimate Kidney Transplant Smoothie Recipes Cookbook" is an amazing and priceless tool for everyone who has had a kidney transplant or is trying to enhance their kidney health. This book is a veritable gold mine of delicious and nutritious smoothie recipes created especially to meet the particular dietary requirements of kidney transplant recipients. This cookbook guarantees that patients may enjoy tasty, nutrient-rich smoothies without sacrificing their health by emphasizing tastes and ingredients that are good for their kidneys.

This cookbook's recipes are proof of the potency of healthful components combined with inventive flavor combinations. The guidebook offers a wide variety of recipes that suit a variety of palates, from the spicy and refreshing Pineapple Mint Refresher to the rich and creamy Avocado Banana Smoothie. Fresh fruits, vegetables, and low-sodium, low-potassium components are prioritized to make sure that every smoothie not only satisfies palates but also promotes kidney health.

Moreover, **"The Ultimate Kidney Transplant Smoothie Recipes Cookbook"** provides a thorough guide for anyone navigating the difficult seas of post-transplant diet; it is more than simply a cookbook. The book offers insightful advice, helpful hints, and thorough descriptions of the advantages of every component to help readers make well-informed dietary decisions. Giving people the tools to take control of their health and well-being, it provides a clear road map for sustaining a healthy diet and enough water after kidney transplantation.

In conclusion, this cookbook is a lifeline for those seeking to emphasize their renal health and kidney transplant patients; it's more than simply a compilation of recipes. It provides a delicious method to follow dietary limitations without compromising flavor, acting as a lifeline for those navigating the challenges of post-transplant nutrition. **"The Ultimate Kidney Transplant Smoothie Recipes Cookbook"** is a culinary treasure that is a need for anybody who wants to enjoy the process of improving their kidney health in addition to nourishing their body.

www.ingramcontent.com/pod-product-compliance
Lightning Source LLC
Chambersburg PA
CBHW050518290526
45786CB00007B/2610